# EASY GUIDE TO INTERMITTENT FASTING

## MELISSA BENNETT

### 2018

You can also purchase my previous books:

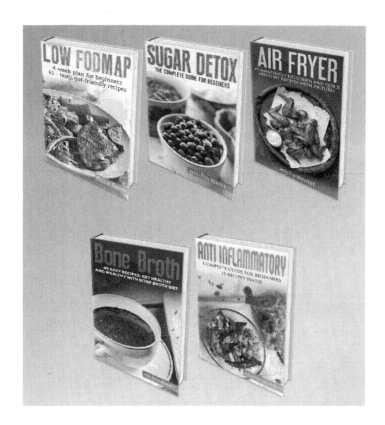

LowFODMAP Diet -
https://www.amazon.com/gp/product/B075FD1TLT
Sugar Detox -
https://www.amazon.com/gp/product/B075FTZPH5
Air Fryer -
https://www.amazon.com/gp/product/B074NGB3QZ
Bone Broth -
https://www.amazon.com/gp/product/B074P4M9LR
Anti-Inflammatory Diet -
https://www.amazon.com/gp/product/B07819K2F8

# Table of Contents

# Introduction

## What Is Intermittent Fasting?

Intermittent fasting refers to a dieting regime that allows you to manage the periods of time you eat and fast within the 24-hour span of a day. It does not dictate the type of food you are expected to consume, it, however, outlines when (time) you can consume them.

Multiple intermittent fasting approaches are available today; the process is centered around dividing your days into consecutive periods of fasting or eating. As humans, the body's natural inclination is to fast while we sleep. To facilitate the process of intermittent fasting simply prolonging your fast after you have awakened.

This can be achieved by eliminating breakfast from your diet. This would now indicate that your first meal would be scheduled for midday and your last at approximately 8 pm.

This popular intermittent approach is known as the 16/8 method. It minimizes your total eating period to 8 hours and extends your fasting period to 16 hours per day.

During the fasting period it is acceptable to intake non-caloric supplements and beverages, this helps to reduce the hunger impulse that some may have. During the initial period "hunger" poses an issue because your body is learning to adjust.

Depending on your body can manage some forms of intermittent fasting will allow you small portions of low-calorie foods during the fasting period. Regardless of how tedious this process sounds, it is quite simple, and the reported benefits are superb.

# Brief History of Fasting

Fasting is a tried and proven heirloom that has withstood not only time but cultures and religions. Fasting is used to aid multiple health conditions including Osteoporosis, improved immune health, weight loss, concentration, and Alzheimer's. Throughout history, fasting has been considered one of the most effective healing tradition.

Fasting is always a controversial topic as people automatically associate the process with starvation. When in fact the two methods are at the other end of the spectrum. The fasting process is planned and controlled while starvation is an uncontrolled occurrence. Starving people are uncertain of their meals or even the means of proving that meal. Fasting, however, is a commitment one act on for either health, spiritual or cleansing purposes. The two concepts must not be compared with each other because the fasting process can be undertaken for a determined period which can span form as long as a one day to months.

Across the world, fasting is distinguished as one of the best traditional practices for healing. Hippocrates of Cos coined the concept of contemporary medicine. His diagnosis was usually remedied with the consumption of apple cider vinegar or the practice of fasting. He quotes, "To eat when one is sick, is to feed that illness." Plutarch another ancient Greek writer/historian voiced a similar sentiment. Quoting, "Instead of using medicine, it's better to fast." Other Greek philosophers such as Plato and Aristotle (his apprentice) were also advocates of the fasting process.

Ancient Greeks observed that nature and our natural surroundings often mirrored our behavioral patterns and actions. You may be able to relate to instances when you are sick, and you immediately lose your appetite. The same trend is noticeable in animals when they are ill. This is the notion behind the phrase 'physician within,' this automatic response our bodies humans and animals alike trigger when we are not in good health. Think back to the last time you were sick, what was the last thing on your agenda? Eating right, which suggests that our anatomy is wired to combat illness through the method of fasting.

It was perceived that fasting improves cognitive functions abilities. Try to think back on your Thanksgiving meals. When you are enjoying your turkey, collard greens, macaroni and cheese, roasted corn, potatoes and all the other goodies that are jam packed on your dinner plate. How do you generally feel afterwards? Are you filled with energy or are you more lethargic, and mentally tired? You usually feel tired, right? This happens due to the fact that some of the blood flow that is generally sent to the brain is rerouted to the digestive system to help your body process the massive shipment of food that you just sent its way. In this state, you would be said to be in a 'food coma.'

Today most if not all religious groups practice fasting as a part of their spiritual journey. The therapeutic benefits of fasting were not only subject to spiritual gains but mental and physical ones also. The benefits of fasting are portrayed in the teachings of many prophets including   Jesus Christ, Muhammed, and Buddha who had a mutual notion of the healing effects of fasting. This spiritual journey often represents a period of purification and atonement; fasting represents spiritual restoration which allows individuals to shed their depravities and strengthen their commitment. Throughout varying cultures and religions, the advancement of fasting was developed primarily to suite their individual beliefs and practices. The practice is not intended to harm the individual carrying out the act but instead reinvigorate their body mind and spirit.

As a Buddhist, you generally consume food primarily in the morning, as many of the followers would be on fasting from midday until meal time the following morning. They also engaged in a number of water fasts (only consuming water) for days, and in some cases weeks. Christians of the Greek

Orthodox era also followed a variety of fasts that engulfed up to 200 days out of each year.

Fasting has also been an important factor in the Muslim community, particularly in the holy month of Ramadan, where the followers are expected to fast from sunrise to sunset daily. It is also important to note that the prophet Muhammad encouraged fasting as frequent as twice weekly on Mondays and Thursdays. However, the month of Ramadan is by far the most popular reference point when it comes to fasting in Islam. During this time all food and drink are forbidden until after sunset each day. Surprisingly studies have shown that though they go so many hours without eating their daily caloric intake tend to peak significantly during Ramadan. This is suspected to be due to 'binge - eating' during the hours that after sunset, and before sunrise that food is actually permitted which reverses any nutritional benefit the fasting period could have had on their bodies.

It's therefore clear that the idea behind fasting has existed for years, and as known to serve various purposes throughout various walks of life for both nutritional, and spiritual benefits. Fasting, over the years, has continued to evolve and is now a powerful tool used to assist in achieving a healthier, and more wholesome life.

## How Intermittent Fasting Work

The background and history of fasting have provided an understanding of the process. Let's delve into the "meat of the matter" providing you with some insight on why and how Intermittent Fasting should be considered.

Intermittent Fasting enables you to structure and work towards your aspirations. for example, weight loss, it is observed that the fewer calories consumed are correlated to weigh loss. During the period of your fast, the caloric intake is significantly reduced, because the window in time for eating has also reduced. It encourages improved insulin adaptability and increased growth hormone secretion, two vital components for weight loss and muscle gain. This practice will help you to not only lose weight but maintain your weight which is the road towards your goal.

During the process, you will realize how everything comes into perspective. You will realize that it is not only your goal of weight loss is achieved but all your other objectives as you see your daily tasks and behaviors become simpler. The process eliminates the need for meal preparations (the what, when and where to eat). Which could also inevitably cause you to save more from your reduced diet.

You now have the time to focus on other activities rather than contemplating on three or more meals per day, with the 16/8 method you are only required to prepare two meals. This method now allows you to enjoy bigger servings making your stomach and taste buds replete while simultaneously consuming fewer calories. Now, let's recap instead of breaking multiple times a day to eat you save a considerable amount of time and energy. Overall reducing associated cost clean-up and travel.

# Chapter 1 - Advantages of Intermittent Fasting

## 1. Encourages Weight Loss

The most profound advantage of intermittent fasting is due to how it boosts your body's capacity to burn fat and help individuals to maintain their weight and build a better physique. Intermittent fasting is considered to be more adaptable that most dieting strategies because it eliminates the factors of you having to track the number of calories per meal.

Intermittent fasting essentially forces your body to exhaust fat it had previously stored for energy, this process then increases the fat burning process which in turn improves weight loss because your body uses sugar (glucose) which is the primary source for our body's energy when you eat, it then stores what is not absorbed in your liver, and muscles as glycogen.

When our body is deprived of a constant glucose supply, it is forced to break down the reserves of glycogen and use it as a source fuel. After which your body will look for a new source of energy (generally your fat cells). These fat cells with then are broken down to help your body produce energy.

## 2. Assists in Regulating Blood Sugar

When carbohydrates are consumed the body converts it to sugar (glucose) in the bloodstream. Insulin is the hormone responsible for transferring glucose from the bloodstream into cells to be used as an energy source.

When the body suffers from ailments such as diabetes, it fails to produce insulin properly which causes elevated levels of glucose in the bloodstream (diabetes). This then leaves the body suffering from complications such as thirst, frequent urination, and fatigue.

Analysis of intermittent fasting has revealed findings that indicate your body improves from the process as it regulates your blood sugar levels, stopping spikes and crashes.

## 3.Takes Care of Your Heart

One of the most profound intermittent fasting advantages is the effect it has on the heart. Findings have indicated that the process has correlated with reduced heart disease complications.

A study of the process showcased the vast influence fasting had on factors directly related to heart health. They observed increased levels good HDL cholesterol and a decrease in bad LDL cholesterol and triglyceride levels.

An animal study reviewed in the Nutritional Biochemistry Journal showed that IMF (intermittent fasting) resulted in a spike in adiponectin levels. The protein that aids the processing of sugars is called Adiponectin; They are said to be defensive in preventing cardiac arrest, and heart diseases. One of the studies on rats noticed that the ones who fasted were 66% likelier to survive a heart attack than the ones on a regular diet.

## 4. Lessens Inflammation Levels

Inflammation is the bodies response to an infection or injury. Chronic inflammation, however, may result in chronic disease. Researchers have determined that inflammation can be linked to chronic conditions such as obesity, diabetes, heart disease and cancer.

A study of 50 individuals partaking in Ramadan was released in the Nutrition Research journal. The findings indicated that the levels of some inflammation markers in the participants decreased during the fasting. In 2015 a separate study revealed that longer spans of night fasting were directly correlated to decreased markers of inflammation.

It has been noted that more in-depth studies are needed in the area, but the available studies have uncovered enough evidence to determine that intermittent fasting could help with the reduction of inflammation and other chronic diseases.

## 5. Protects the Brain

intermittent fasting has not only been proven to improve your chances of chronic diseases such as heart disease, diabetes, and obesity. further studies into intermittent fasting has indicated that it could possibly protect the health of your brain

An animal study revealed that intermittent fasting improved cognitive functions and provided protected against changes in memory and learning function when compared to a controlled group.

Additionally, researchers have noted that anti-inflammatory effects of intermittent fasting can enhance your brain functions which can reduce the progress of diseases like Parkinson's, Alzheimer's, and dementia.

## 6. Reduces Hunger Surges

The hormone responsible for controlling hunger is called Leptin. It is produced when your fat cells signal sends a signal to our body telling it to stop eating. The level of leptin in the body determines hunger. When the levels drop your body feels hunger, and they rise you feel full.

Individuals who are obese usually have higher levels of leptin in their bodies this occurs because the production of this hormone is primary in the body's fat cells. If he body produces an excess amount of leptin, it can make the body resistant to signals that notify the body to stop eating.

A study of 80 individuals whose leptin levels were measured while on intermittent fasting revealed that the hormone levels became lower at night which means they tend to get hungrier at night. This indicates that eating throughout the day and fasting at night could translate to reduced hunger urges leading to further weight loss.

# Chapter 2 – Precautions

As with anything in life, intermittent fasting, though severely beneficial to your health, also has its share of drawbacks. As such it may not be as beneficial to certain people. Here are a few precautions to keep in mind when considering intermittent fasting (IMF).

## 1.   Check your blood sugar levels before starting IMF

It is important that you take the time to check on your blood sugar before deciding to consider intermittent fasting. Whether you suffer low blood sugar levels or diabetes, eating regularly is a vital part of remaining healthy. Due to this, going long periods without eating can possibly lead to drastically low blood sugar levels that may result in dangerous health complications such as fatigue, shakiness, and heart palpitations. As such it is important that you consult your doctor before diving into intermittent fasting to see if it is right for you.

## 2. Examine your eating history

It is recommended that you avoid IMF if you have suffered from eating disorder in the past. Regardless of when it was, whether it was when you were a teen or recently in your adult years, not eating for long periods can possibly trigger symptoms of unhealthy eating and push you back in a negative space.

## 3. Consider your age.

Children and teenagers are advised to avoid doing intermittent fasting. As a child, your main concern should be looking towards a healthy and safe future. As such, there would really be no need for them to go on extremely long fasts. Instead, have them focus on hitting their suggested nutritional targets each day.

## 4. Avoid when sick

When you are sick, your body needs to get a steady nutrient stream in order to heal as such undergoing an intermittent fast while sick can possibly slow down the healing process.

## 5. IMF may be problematic in women

When it comes to IMF, there is a lot of factors for women to consider. Let's start with the obvious. Pregnant, or lactating women should avoid IMF as by limiting the number of times you eat you would also be placing a limit on the number of nutrients you are providing for your unborn child. So instead of fasting, consider eating a balanced diet which will give you the adequate number of nutrients needed to maintain a healthy pregnancy.

Now for the part that may be less obvious. Long term intermittent fasting may lead to hormonal issues which may result in issues with weight control, regulating menstruation cycles, pregnancy, menopause, puberty, hair growth, and skin complexion to name a few. As such if you opt to do intermittent fasting, consider doing it just a few days for the week, instead of making it a daily routine.

## 6. Avoid with gallbladder issues

There is a possibility that fasting can increase the risks associated with gallbladder problems. Due to this if you have a history of gallstone disease it may not be wise to do IMF.

## 7. IMF can affect thyroid

As mentioned before, intermittent fasting can alter hormones, which includes the thyroid regulating hormones. As such if you have a history of thyroid issues this may not be the plan for you.

## 8. If you are a gym junkie avoid IMF

That's right! Despite all the misconceptions you hear you have to be careful if you are considering intermittent fasting a gym junkie. People who are extremely active can throw their bodies into shock while intermittent fasting as your body needs nutrients before working out and after to replenish. So, if you do choose to partake in intermittent fasting while physically active, try to take it easy in the gym on the days you are fasting and ensure that you stay hydrated. However, if you plan a fast that is more than 72 hours, it is strongly advised that you limit your physical activity.

# Chapter 3 – Types of Intermittent Fasting

Now that we have explored a bit of the history of intermittent fasting, advantages, and precautions, let's dive in a bit more exploring some of the different categories of fasting.

## 1. The Twelve-Hour Fast

The first category we will explore is the Twelve Hour Fast. As the name suggests, it involves fasting for 12 consecutive hours in a day. I know it sounds difficult, but it's honestly not. So, are you ready to go fasting for a full twelve hours?

Before you start panicking, stop to really think it. The average sleeps for between 7 – 9 hours daily which means there would just be an additional 3 – 5 hours that you would need to fast. That's right! The hours that you are sleeping counts towards your fast. So, thinking of a typical day, this may even be close to the routine you currently have.

A typical day on a twelve-hour fast plan would involve waking up at around 7AM to enjoy a full meal for breakfast, then dinner at 7PM as the final meal of the day. Between this time, the best thing you can do is try to stay busy. When your mind is occupied your body tends to forget about food. So, if you work the typical hours of 9 – 5 then this would be the perfect opportunity to engulf yourself in work. Another way to make the hours speed by is to try and get some sleep.

**How can you be sure it works?**

This twelve-hour fast plan was initially tested in a study with four groups of mice. The study was to evaluate how weight loss was affected when using this variation of intermittent fasting versus eating normally. The four different groups of mice were then fed the same number of calories each day, allowing them to eat at different intervals. The two groups that stood out in terms of results were the one that was tested on the 12-hour intermittent fast and the group that ate whenever they wanted to.

The group that ate during a 12-hour window and fasted for the remaining 12 experienced the most successful rate of weight loss, as the more rigid they were with this structure, the more they lost. On the other hand, the group that was allowed to eat at random hours of the day actually gained weight even though both groups consumed the same number of calories. From these results, the researchers were able to safely conclude that weight loss was more efficient when following a rigid intermittent fasting plan.

**Who is this plan recommended for?**

Just about anyone can experience success in the twelve- hour fast plan, however, it is generally recommended to people who are new to the world of intermittent fasting. This is largely due to the fact that this is extremely similar to the hours of an average diet outside a fast, making it easy to adjust to. The idea is to stick to the recommended number of calories related to a healthy diet for your BMI range in the specific time window, then fasting for the remaining hours to allow your body to convert energy from fat cells. As soon as you get used to the idea of the science behind intermittent fasting you can start exploring other fasting categories.

## 2. The Eight Hour Window (16/8 Protocol)

If you have been using the twelve – hour fast and wanted to take your fasting result up to another level then the eight-hour window plan, also known as the 16/8 protocol, may be the category for you. Now, it is important that you understand that this plan will be even more rigid, and possibly harder for you to maintain than the twelve-hour plan. However, if you are able

18

to make the push and follow the plan than your reward will be unforgettable.

As the name suggests, this plan involves eating your recommended daily caloric dose with an eight-hour window then fasting for the remaining sixteen hours of the day. A prime example of this would be a person who eats their first meal at noon then their final meal for that day at 8PM. This cycle would then be repeated each day that you remain on this intermittent fasting plan. This plan is a bit trickier to maintain, but it is just as effective as the initial twelve-hour, and as even been scientifically proven to aid in the prevention of obesity, diabetes, and liver disease.

**Selecting the best hours to eat**

You will have to figure out the best eating window for you based on your current lifestyle. However, here are a few of the popular windows of the eight-hour window plan that you can use as a base to create your own:

> Have your first meal at 7AM, consume no more food, and begin your fast at 3pm
> Have your first meal at 11AM, consume no more food, and begin your fast at 7pm
> Have your first meal at 2PM, consume no more food, and begin your fast at 10pm
> Have your first meal at 6PM, consume no more food, and begin your fast at 2AM.

Only you can select the best plan for you. It's always better to select hours that already ties in to your current schedule as this will make it easier for you to stick with your selection for the long haul. Remember structure, and organization breathes success.

## 3. The 5:2 Plan

The next category we will explore is a bit different from the ones we have been through. This plan focuses on the variation of 'fasting days' rather than 'fasting hours.' Essentially, the plan allows you to eat normally for 5 days of the week and depleting your caloric intake to only 25% of your calorie needs for the remaining 2 days of the week.

Eating normally, however, does not mean 5 days filled with fried chicken, burger, and pizza as what you eat in these 5 days will make or break the number you see on the scale each week. Instead, try to maintain a healthy, and balanced diet at all times.

**How to eat on the two 'fasting days'?**

Unlike the other fasting plans covered this plan as no actual time that you are forced to restrain from food. Though the days are called "fasting days" you are still required to eat. What you consume, however, would be different than the other days as your calories allowance is significantly smaller.

There are two popular meal patterns that are used for "fasting days." These are:

> ➢ Consuming 3 small meals for the day: a small breakfast, small lunch or snack, and small dinner OR
> ➢ Skipping a meal and only eating 2 slightly larger meals throughout the day.

It is important that your calorie allowance is used wisely, especially on these days as the allowance is generally as low as 600 calories per fasting day for men, and 500 calories per fasting day for women. Focus on low calorie foods that are high in protein, high in fiber and extremely nutritious.

**The following is a list of foods that can be considered for your fasting days:**

- ✓ Large vegetable portions
- ✓ Berries, and organic yogurt
- ✓ Eggs
- ✓ Fish (preferably grilled)
- ✓ Lean meat (preferably grilled)
- ✓ Cauliflower rice
- ✓ Vegetable soups
- ✓ Low-calorie ramen
- ✓ Coffee (preferably black)
- ✓ Tea (unsweetened or with natural low-calorie sweetener)
- ✓ Water

Bear in mind; these are all just suggestions you feel to come up with your own low-calorie selections. So, mix, and match to find the best meal plan for you on these 2 days. As long as you adhere to the calorie restriction, and make your choices with nutritional value in mind, you will be fine.

## 4. Alternate-Day Fasting

Like the 5:2 plan, alternative day fasting involves the variation of "fasting days," and "feeding days." As the names suggest, this plan allows you to eat 'normally' on one day, depleting your caloric intake to only 25% of your calorie needs the next day, then repeating to create a, eating cycle.

As expected you want to keep your meals nutritional, and low calories on your "fast days" getting your calories mainly from healthy fats, lean protein, and vegetables. Avoid foods that are high in starch and any product with refined sugars. Eating like this will ensure that you achieve the maximum level of weight loss.

**Benefits of the Alternate Day Fasting Plan**

The alternate-day fasting plan has been proven to provide a wide array of benefits including:

> ➢ Increasing the rate of weight loss which in turn combats Obesity
> ➢ Reducing the risk of Type 2 Diabetes
> ➢ Promoting Cardiovascular health
> ➢ Aiding in the regulation of blood pressure levels

The list of benefits could go on, and on as there is no end to what you can achieve when you buckle down, and stick to this plan.

The same can be said of any of the intermittent fasting plans covered in this chapter. So, regardless of the plan, you opt to follow remember that structure, and organization will always be the key to your success. Now it's time to explore a few tips and tricks that will help to keep you motivated along your journey.

# Chapter 4 - Tips, Hacks & Motivation

Are you freaking out? Stop it! Don't do that to yourself! Stop asking yourself if you can fast 9 hours instead of 12 or thinking that just sneaking an apple during your fast is okay. After all, it's an apple, right? What're a few hours, right? Wrong! It's really not about the few hours you shave off or even the apple; it's what it represents. Our bodies are complex machines that learn to adapt with repetition. So, it's not all as harmless or simple as you think it may be. However, it also is nothing to beat yourself up about! Your first step to being successful on this journey is learning to relax.

This diet plan is in no way black, and white. It's okay to eat breakfast one day, then decide not to have breakfast the next. It's all dependent on what you are ultimately trying to achieve. If optimal athletic performance what you are going for then sure a more rigid schedule and diet will be needed, but, failing that … relax! Stop stressing out over minutiae! Simply jump back on the horse and keep on riding towards a healthier you. Perfection is never to be confused for the enemy of 'doing good,' you will have perfect days now, and again but your best will always be good enough even if you don't feel like it. On those days when you honestly find yourself struggling to continue on your journey try making use of one or more of these popular tips, tricks, and hacks for fasting motivation.

## 1. Start Walking

Believe it or not, even low intensity walks can be helpful on those frustrating fasting mornings. These walks can help to put your mind at ease, so you can prepare for the day ahead. Best of all it helps to boost the rate at which your body burns fat. Ideally, you want to take your walks first thing in the morning, but if you can't, another time of day will work as well.

## 2. Don't Push Too Hard on Fasting Days

If you choose to work out on the days that you fast, it will be vital that you listen to what your body is saying to you. Exercising can be difficult while fasting as you tend to get feelings of light headedness, and a lack of stamina to drive performance. If you find that you begin to experience this ensure that you are fully hydrated and that while in your 'feeding windows' you are hitting the correct number of calories that you should be for your specific body mass index. If you are, evaluate what it is that you are eating to hit this caloric mark. You want to ensure that most your calories are coming from healthy fats, and protein.

## 3. Be Prepare for Possible Breakfast Criticism

There may be a few run ins with 'naysayers' or even family members that are full on breakfast eaters and believe that they should convince you to habitually do the same. This is all due to they will we were all raised. So many of us have grown up hearing that "Breakfast is the most important meal of the day." Due to this, there are so many people that just will not understand why you have decided to skip breakfast and begin eating at lunch time, for example, but when this happens, stand your ground and reminding yourself of the science behind that very statement.

The word 'breakfast' is the term used to identify the first meal of the day, the meal that 'breaks the fast.' Although it has over the years become the norm to be the morning meal it does not particularly have to be eaten in the morning. So, remind yourself of this the next time you find yourself considering the words of your 'naysayers.'

## 4. Keep Your Mind Occupied

Try to keep yourself busy. If you have not figured it out as yet, you will soon find out that as soon as your brain has slowed down with nothing to think about, it will start to occupy your mind with thoughts of hunger. Instead, try to ensure that your fasting windows are strategically planned around your busier periods, and if you can't schedule it around your general sleeping time.

## 5. Test Yourself with Zero Calorie Beverages

That's right; you are allowed to drink more than water during your fating windows. Beverages with zero calories are also acceptable. However, the only way to be 100% certain that it is a zero-calorie drink is to make it from scratch in your own kitchen. These are generally simple to whip up and can include:

- ✓ Herbal teas
- ✓ Herb infused waters
- ✓ Iced tea (sugar free)
- ✓ And of course, water.

## 6. Tweak Your Diet to Suit You

It's important that you understand that everybody is different. Your specific goals may be different from even your spouse, and as such will need to listen to your body and tweak your diet, and caloric needs accordingly. Don't beat yourself up if your find that you need to start out with larger portions that someone else. Never deprive yourself, instead make small changes gradually until you are able to comfortably get to where you need to be.

## 7. Maintain a Realistic Mindset

As much as we would like to believe that you will be the next great miracle of intermittent fasting, it is better to keep your expectations as realistic as possible. Sure, intermittent fasting, if done correctly, has the potential to assist you in your weight loss journey, increase your body's sensitivity to insulin, and regulate the rate in which your body secretes growth hormones, which are all wonderful benefits. However, it is important that you also keep in mind that intermittent fasting is just one aspect of the many things you will need to adjust in your life to achieve success in your body's overall health. You will also need to adjust your overall level of activity, amount of sleep, stress levels and it will take time.

# Chapter 5 – Sample Meal Plan for Fasting Days

Fantastic job at getting through all that information! I know it was a mouthful, but it was vital that you equipped yourself with a clear understanding of the history, categories, and struggles associated with the diet plan before diving directly into it. So, now that you are ready to begin, here is a **sample 7-day meal** plan perfect for the **<u>Fasting Days</u>** while on the **5:2 Plan or Alternate Day Fasting** that you can use as a base when creating your very own plan to follow.

Fast Day 1 - Breakfast: Oats Porridge

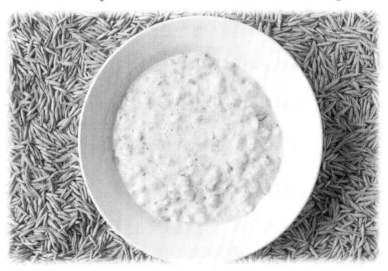

*Serves: 1*

**Time: 5 mins**

**Ingredients:**

Quaker Oats (40g)

Milk (180 ml, 1%)

## Directions:

Add your milk to a small saucepan over medium heat, and allow to come to a boil, while stirring. Add oats, stir, and lower your heat so that the mixture just simmers. Allow to simmer, stirring occasionally, until your milk becomes mostly absorbed (about 2 additional minutes).

## Nutritional Information per Serving:

Calories: 255; Total Fat: 9 g; Carbs: 35 g; Protein: 12.6 g

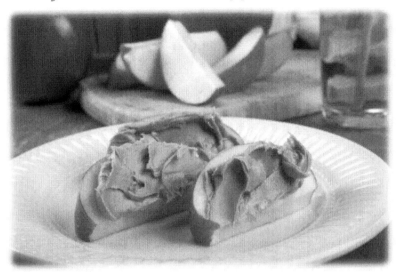

*Serves: 1*

**Time: 5 mins**

**Ingredients:**

Apple (2, Granny Smith)

Almond Butter (2 tbsp.)

**Directions:**

Prepare your apple, by breaking the stem then slicing to discard the seeds and core. Slice your apples into thin slices, and lay them flat on a serving plate. Top with drizzles of almond butter, and enjoy!

**Nutritional Information per Serving:**

Calories: 250; Total Fat: 24 g; Carbs: 50 g; Protein: 2 g

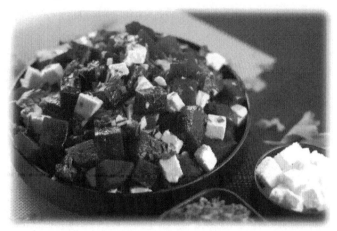

***Serves: 1***

**Time: 5 mins**

**Ingredients:**

Beetroot (50 grams, roasted)

Spinach (60 grams)

Feta (30 grams)

Lemon juice (1 tsp.)

**Directions:**

Using gloves, cut your beetroot into wedges then add to a large bowl. Add all your remaining ingredients, and toss to combine. Enjoy!

**Nutritional Information per Serving:**

Calories: 125; Total Fat: 7 g; Carbs: 8 g; Protein: 7 g

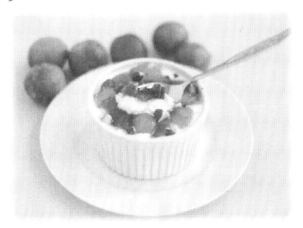

***Serves: 1***

**Time: 30 mins**

**Ingredients:**

Yogurt (100 grams, low fat)

Plums (2, halved)

Honey (1 tsp.)

**Directions:**

Set your oven to preheat to 400 degrees F, and prepare a baking sheet by lining with aluminum foil, and lightly greasing with olive oil. Add your plums, and honey to a medium bowl, and stir to fully coat. Transfer your honey coated plums to your baking sheet, and set to roast until juicy, and soft (about 15 minutes). Remove from heat, and allow to cool slightly. Add your yogurt to a serving bowl, then top with roasted plum. Drizzle with plum juices, and serve.

**Nutritional Information per Serving:**

Calories: 145; Total Fat: 8 g; Carbs: 10 g; Protein: 10 g

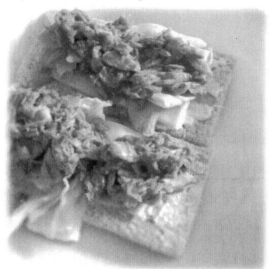

*Serves: 1*

**Time: 5 mins**

**Ingredients:**

Ryvita crackerbreads (2)

Tuna salad (60 grams)

Arugula (70 grams)

Black pepper (1 tsp, cracked)

**Directions:**

Lay your Ryvita crackerbreads flat on a serving plate. Top with tuna salad, and argula. Season with black pepper and serve.

**Nutritional Information per Serving:**

Calories: 253; Total Fat: 3 g; Carbs: 8 g; Protein: 50 g

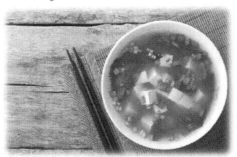

*Serves: 2*

**Time: 15 mins**

**Ingredients:**

Water (4 cups)

Green chard (1/2 cup, chopped)

Green Onion (1/2 cup, chopped)

Tofu (1/4 cup, firm, cubed)

Miso (3 tbsp., white, paste)

Nori (2 sheets, thinly sliced)

**Directions:**

Set a medium saucepan with water, over medium heat, and allow to rise to a low simmer. Add nori then continue simmering for about 7 minutes. Add miso in a small bowl with a bit of the water from the pot, and whisk to form a smooth paste. Add to saucepan, stir, then add all your remaining ingredients. Allow to cook for another 6 or so minutes. Serve.

**Nutritional Information per Serving:**

Calories: 88; Total Fat: 2 g; Carbs: 9 g; Protein: 7 g;

# Fast Day 3 - Breakfast: Soft boiled Egg and Asparagus

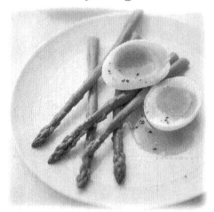

**Serves: 1**

**Time: 15 mins**

**Ingredients:**

Egg (1 large)

Asparagus (5 long, peeled, trimmed)

Salt and pepper (to taste)

**Directions:**

Set a large saucepan with salted water over high heat, and allow to come to a boil. Add e asparagus and cook until fork tender (about 5 min). Add your egg to the saucepan at the same time, and allow to cook for 3 minutes. Set an egg cup with egg on a serving plate and serve alongside asparagus, salt, and pepper.

**Nutritional Information per Serving:**

Calories: 90; Total Fat: 5 g; Carbs: 4 g; Protein: 8.5 g;

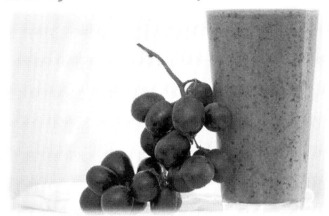

*Serves: 1*

**Time: 5 mins**

**Ingredients:**

Grapes (1 cup)

Spinach (1 cup)

Banana (1/2)

Goji berries (1 tbsp.)

Pea protein blend (1 tbsp.)

Orange juice (2 tbsp.)

Almond milk (1½ cups)

**Directions:**

Add all your ingredients to a blender, and process until smooth. Transfer to a serving glass, and enjoy!

**Nutritional Information per Serving:**
Calories:292.3; Total Fat: 5.2g; Carbs:54.5g; Protein: 12.5g

# Fast Day 3 - Dinner: Turkey Burgers with Corn

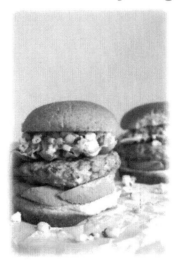

*Serves: 1*

**Time: 5 mins**

**Ingredients:**

Burger mix:

Turkey mince (111g)

Egg (1, beaten)

Spring onion (1 tbsp., chopped)

Garlic (1 clove, minced)

Chili Pepper (1/2 tsp, ground)

Corn on the cob (1, medium, warmed)

**Directions:**

Add all your burger ingredients to a large bowl, and gently massage to combine. Set to marinate in the refrigerator for at least 30 minutes. Split your mixture evenly in half, and form into 2 burger patties. Cook on a preheated grill until fully cooked (about 5 min per side). Serve alongside corn on the cob.

**Nutritional Information per Serving:**

Calories: 328; Total Fat: 17 g; Carbs: 30 g; Protein: 19 g;

# Fast Day 4 - Breakfast: Avocado Belvita Breakfast Biscuits

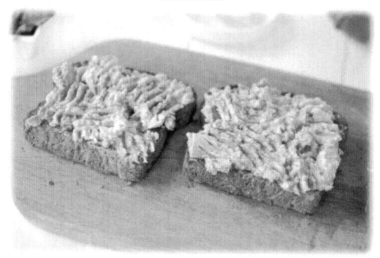

***Serves: 1***

**Time: 5 mins**

**Ingredients:**

Belvita Breakfast Biscuits (4, blueberry)

Avocado (100 grams, mashed)

Salt, and pepper (to taste)

**Directions**

Lay your biscuits flat on a serving plate, and top with mashed avocado. Season to taste, and serve.

**Nutritional Information per Serving:**

Calories: 388; Total Fat: 24g; Carbs: 48g; Protein: 12g;

# Fast Day 4 - Lunch: Mango Chia Pudding

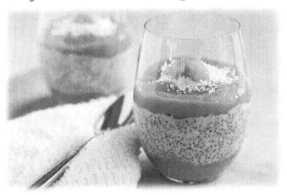

*Serves: 6*

**Time: 2 hours 10 mins**

**Ingredients:**

Flax milk (1 ½ cups, coconut flavored)

Large mango (1, cut into chunks)

Vanilla extract (1 tsp.)

Tea salt (1/8 tsp.)

Chia seed (7 tbs.)

Cinnamon (3 tbs.)

**Directions:**

Add all ingredients in a blender and blend until the ingredients are combined and smooth. Put the mixture into a bowl and it in the fridge for 2 hours or until it thickens.

Serve and enjoy!

**Nutritional Information per Serving:**

Calories: 159; Total Fat: 10g; Carbs:18g; Protein:4g

# Fast Day 4 - Dinner: Roasted Vegetables with Balsamic Glaze

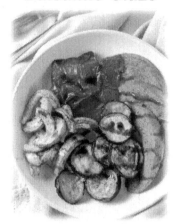

*Serves: 1*

**Time: 40 mins**

**Ingredients:**

Courgette (1/2)

Aubergine (1/2)

Butternut squash (1/2)

Red pepper (1/2)

Balsamic vinegar (2 tbsp.)

Lemon Juice (1 tsp.)

**Directions:**

Set oven to preheat to 425 degrees F, and prepare a baking sheet by lining with aluminum foil. Add all your ingredients to a large bowl, and toss to combine. Transfer to the prepped baking sheet, and set to roast for about 30 minutes (vegetables should be caramelized, yet tender). Serve.

**Nutritional Information per Serving:**

Calories: 261; Total Fat: 2 g; Carbs: 57 g; Protein: 13 g;

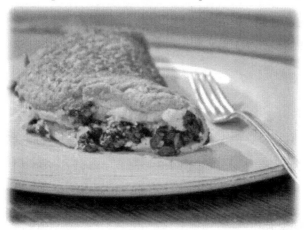

*Serves: 1*

**Time: 10 mins**

**Ingredients:**

Eggs (2)

spinach leaves (60 grams)

Salt and pepper (to taste)

**Directions:**

Add your eggs and spinach together in a medium bowl, season with salt, and pepper and whisk to combine. Set a lightly greased skillet over medium heat, and allow to get hot. Add egg mixture, once hot, and cook until egg begins to set (about 3 min). Flip your egg over halfway to form an omelet, and continue to cook until fully set (about another 2 mins). Enjoy!

**Nutritional Information per Serving:**

Calories: 161; Total Fat: 10 g; Carbs: 6 g; Protein: 13 g

# Fast Day 5 – Lunch: Edamame Beans

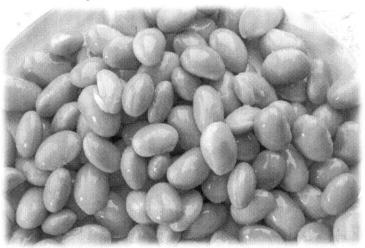

*Serves: 1*

**Time: 7 mins**

**Ingredients:**

Edamame beans (60 grams)

Rock salt – (1 tsp.)

**Directions:**

Set a medium saucepan with salted water over high heat, and allow to come to a boil. Once boiling, add edamame beans and cook until tender (about 5 min). Drain, and carefully drop beans out of pods into a medium bowl. Add rock salt and toss to evenly coat. Enjoy!

**Nutritional Information per Serving:**

Calories: 84; Total Fat: 4 g; Carbs: 7 g; Protein: 8 g;

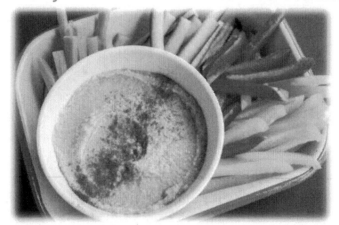

*Serves: 1*

**Time: 5 mins**

**Ingredients:**

Hummus (40 grams)

Carrots (3 jumbo, cut into small sticks)

Cucumber (1/2 cup, cut into small sticks)

Red Bell Pepper (1/2 cup, cut into small sticks)

**Directions:**

Add your hummus to a small bowl, and set in the center of a serving plate. Add your veggies around the hummus, and enjoy!

**Nutritional Information per Serving:**

Calories: 175; Total Fat: 4.3 g; Carbs: 31 g; Protein: 6 g;

# Fast Day 6 – Breakfast: Banana Low-Fat Yogurt

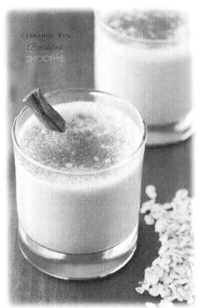

***Serves: 1***

**Time: 5 mins**

**Ingredients:**

Yogurt (100 grams, low – fat)

Banana (1)

Cinnamon (1/4 tsp.)

**Directions:**

Combine all your ingredients in your blender, and process until smooth. Enjoy!

**Nutritional Information per Serving:**

Calories: 177; Total Fat: 2.2 g; Carbs: 36.2 g; Protein: 7 g;

# Fast Day 6 – Curried Carrot, Sweet Potato, and Ginger Soup

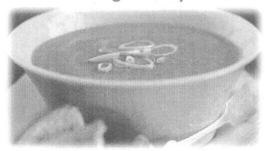

*Serves: 3*

**Time: 35min**

**Ingredients:**

Extra Virgin Olive Oil (2 tsp.)

Shallots (½ cup, chopped)

Sweet Potato (3 cups, peeled, cubed)

Carrots (1½ cup, peeled, sliced)

**Directions:**

Place a saucepan with your oil on medium heat until it just begins to smoke. Add your shallots to the pot and sauté until it becomes tender (should take approximately 2 – 3 min). Add all your prepped vegetables to the shallots, and your curry then allow to cook for another 2 minutes. Pour in your broth and allow it to come to a boil. Once boiling, place the lid on the pot and reduce the heat to low. Allow this mixture to simmer until your vegetables are all tender. Once tender, add salt and pour your soup into a food processor. Pulse until creamy and smooth. Strain, serve and Enjoy.

**Nutritional Information per Serving:**

Calories: 144; Total Fat: 2.3g; Carbs: 27.3g; Protein: 4.1 g;

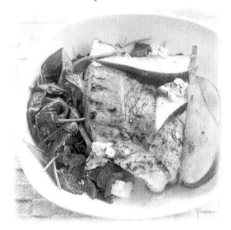

**Serves: 1**

**Time: 45 min.**

**Ingredients:**

Turkey breast (125 grams, cleaned and dried)

Spinach (1 cup, cooked)

Salt, and pepper (1 tsp. each)

**Directions:**

Set your oven to preheat to 400 degrees F, and prepare a baking sheet by lining it with aluminum foil. Lay your turkey breast on the baking sheet, and season with salt, and pepper. Set to bake until turkey breast has been fully cooked (about 30 minutes). Remove from oven and let stand at room temperature for about 5 minutes before serving. Serve alongside reheated spinach.

**Nutritional Information per Serving:**

Calories: 216; Total Fat: 1.2 g; Carbs: 5.5 g; Protein: 42 g

# Fast Day 7 - Breakfast: Apple, Carrot and Ginger Smoothie

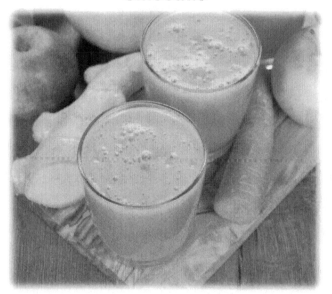

*Serves: 1*

**Time: 5 min.**

**Ingredients:**

Apple (1, cored, chopped)

Carrot (1 jumbo, chopped)

Ginger (1 tbsp., chopped)

**Directions:**

Combine all your ingredients in your blender, and process until smooth.

**Nutritional Information per Serving:**

Calories: 211.2; Total Fat: 1.3 g; Carbs: 54.7 g; Protein: 2.6 g;

# Fast Day 7- Lunch: Blueberries Banana Almond Smoothie

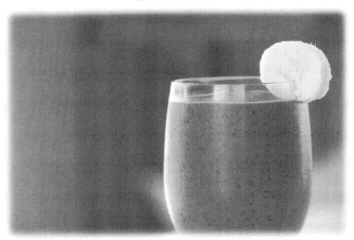

*Serves: 1*

**Time: 5 min.**

**Ingredients:**

Blueberries (200 grams, frozen)

Banana (1, chopped)

Almond milk (1 cup)

**Directions:**

Combine all your ingredients in your blender, and process until smooth.

**Nutritional Information per Serving:**

Calories: 189.1; Total Fat: 4.1g; Carbs: 40.0 g; Protein: 2.7 g

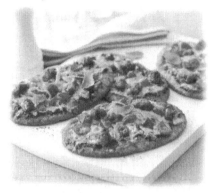

***Serves: 1***

**Time: 10 min.**

**Ingredients:**

Pitta bread (1, whole wheat)

Mozzarella cheese (25 grams, shredded)

Tomato (1, diced)

Herbs (1 tbsp., of your choosing)

Salt and pepper (to taste)

**Directions**

Set your oven to preheat to 400 degrees F, and prepare a baking sheet by lightly greasing with olive oil. Lay your pita on a flat surface. Top with cheese, tomatoes, and herbs, then season with salt, and pepper. Transfer to baking sheet, and set to bake until cheese is melted, and pita slightly golden (about 7 minutes). Enjoy!

**Nutritional Information per Serving:**

Calories: 178; Total Fat: 2 g; Carbs: 36 g; Protein: 5 g;

# Chapter 6 – Sample Meal Plan for Feeding Days

In the past chapter, we explored sample recipes that you can enjoy as is or tweak for your fasting days. Now let's explore a few recipes that you can enjoy while on your normal **feeding days** or while eating normally on the **12 - Hour window plan** or the **16/8 Protocol.**

## Day 1 – Breakfast: Almond Flour Pancakes

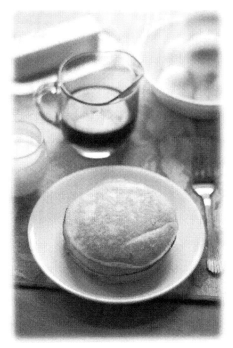

*Serves: 3*

**Time: 20 min**

**Ingredients:**

Almond Flour (1¾ cups)

Baking Powder (1 tsp.)

Tapioca Flour (2 tbsp.)

Salt (1/4 tsp.)

Eggs (2, lightly beaten)

Vanilla Extract (1 tsp.)

Almond Milk (3/4 cup)

## Directions

Add all your wet ingredients to a medium bowl and whisk to combine. Add your dry ingredients and gently mix until fully combined and smooth. Set a skillet on over medium heat and lightly coat with coconut oil. Cook your pancakes (1/4 cup of batter per pancake) for about 4 minutes per side. Serve, and enjoy your favorite pancake syrup on the side.

## Nutritional Information per Serving:

Calories: 123.3; Total Fat: 10.4 g; Carbs: 3.6 g; Protein: 5.5 g;

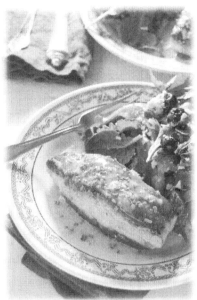

*Serves: 4*

**Time: 20 min**

**Ingredients**

Fish (4, cut into halves e.g Sea Bass)

Black pepper (1/4 teaspoon)

Olive oil (1 tablespoon)

White wine (1/2 cup, dry)

Chives (1 tablespoon, snipped)

Salt (1/4 teaspoon)

Whole wheat flour (3 tablespoons)

Shallots (1/2 cup, diced)

Fish stock (1 cup)

## Directions

Use pepper and salt to season fish. Put flour into a dish and use to coat fish thoroughly. Heat oil in a skillet and cook for 5 minutes on one side until golden. Flip fish and cook for 5 minutes on the other side; remove from heat and put aside. Prepare sauce by heating a skillet and cooking shallots for 2 minutes then add wine and cook for 1 minute until wine reduces by half. Use a spoon to scrape pan. Add broth to skillet and cook for 4 minutes, stir and cook until liquid reduces by half. Add chives and then add fish. Heat thoroughly and serve.

## Nutritional Information per Serving:

Calories: 257; Total Fat: 9 g; Carbs: 26 g; Protein: 26 g;

# Day 1 – Dinner: Smoked BBQ Beans

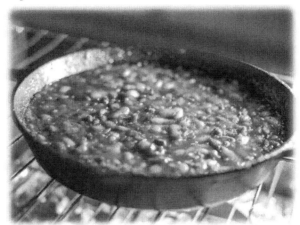

*Serves: 3-4*

**Time: 1 hr.**

**Ingredients:**

Bacon (center cut, 5 slices, chopped)

Yellow Onion (1, chopped)

Garlic Cloves (5, minced)

Jalapeno (1, chopped)

Pinto (1 lb.)

Water (6 Cups)

BBQ Sauce (1 Cup)

Spicy Brown Mustard (2 Tbsp.)

Adobe Sauce (2 Tbsp., from canned Chipotles)

Tabasco Sauce (2 Tbsp., smoked)

Molasses (2 Tbsp.)

Guinness (splash, optional)

Salt (2 Tsp)

Pepper (1 tsp)

## Directions

Prepare your beans (wash, sort, and soak) from overnight. Set your Dutch oven to preheat on the top of the stove. Add bacon to the heated oven and allow to brown until crisp. At this point, add the jalapeno and onions then proceed to sauté until onions become soft. Continue to sauté while you add the garlic. Continue for about a minute. Pour in the beans, and water then cover and allow cooking on low to medium heat for about an hour or until the beans become soft. Add a bit of your preferred BBQ sauce along with the brown sugar, adobo sauce, Tabasco, mustard salt and pepper while stirring well.

Remove the cover and allow simmering until the sauce thickens and the beans become completely cooked (should be about an hour). Serve and enjoy.

## Nutritional Information per Serving:

Calories: 210; Total Fat: 1.5 g; Carbs: 41 g; Protein: 8 g;

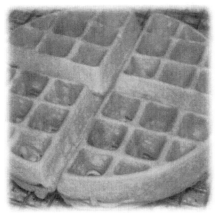

*Serves: 1*

**Time: 20 min**

**Ingredients:**

Coconut flour (1 cups)

Salt (1/4 tsp.)

Baking Soda (1/4 tsp.)

Eggs (4)

Vanilla (1 tsp.)

Honey (2 tbsp.)

Cinnamon (1/4 tsp.)

**Directions**

Add all your wet ingredients to a medium bowl and whisk to combine. Add your dry ingredients and gently mix until fully combined and smooth. Set your waffle iron to get hot, and lightly coat with coconut oil. Cook your waffles (1/4 cup of batter per waffle) for about 5 minutes. Serve, and enjoy with maple syrup.

57

## Nutritional Information per Serving:

Calories: 467.1; Total Fat: 39.3 g; Carbs: 13.2 g; Protein: 15.6 g;

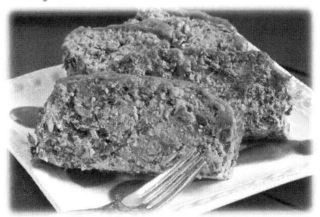

*Serves: 4*

**Time: 1hr. 30min**

**Ingredients**

1 lb. minced beef

¾ cup almond flour

1 egg (beaten)

½ cup ketchup and pica pepper (mixed)

½ cup onion and scallion (chopped finely)

2 tbsp. sweet pepper (chopped)

1 sprig thyme

1 tsp. ea. salt & pepper

**Directions**

Preheat oven to 350 degrees F. Grease a loaf tin or shallow baking dish. Combine all ingredients and mix well. Shake into greased loaf tin or dish. Cover over with foil paper. Bake for 1 hour. Serve hot.

**Nutritional Information per Serving:**

Calories: 285 Total Fat: 14.01 g; Carbs: 10.74 g; Protein: 29.88 g;

# Day 2 – Dinner: Honey Mustard Chicken Drumsticks

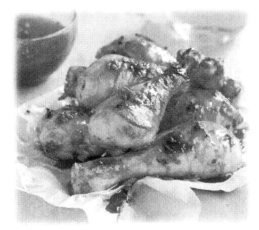

***Serves: 6***

**Time: 1 hr. 30min**

**Ingredients**

3 lbs. drumsticks

4 oz. flour

1 tsp. salt

½ tsp. paprika

1 tsp. white pepper

½ tsp. chicken seasoning

½ cup soft margarine

½ cup honey

½ cup mustard

6 tsp. lime juice

½ tsp. salt

## Directions

Wash and drain drumsticks.  Use a clean cloth or paper towel to dry chicken. In a paper bag, combine salt, almond flour, paprika, chicken seasoning and white pepper. Put chicken in bag and shake vigorously to coat properly. Melt margarine in a baking pan, roll pieces of chicken in melted margarine until all sides are coated.

Fix the chicken pieces, skin side down in the baking pan, packing them close to each other but not overcrowded. Bake at 400 degrees F for 30 minutes.  Turn chicken pieces over and pour on glaze.  Bake for a further 20 minutes or until cooked.  Set aside. Mix all ingredients together and pour over chicken and serve.

## Nutritional Information per Serving:

Calories: 93.3 Total Fat: 2.9 g; Carbs: 3.9 g; Protein: 12.9 g;

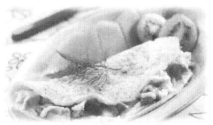

***Serves: 2***

**Time: 10 minutes**

**Ingredients:**

Eggs (4)

Soy Sauce (1¼ tsp.) soy sauce

Arugula (4 tbsps., leaves only)

Red Pepper (1, roasted, sliced into coins)

Pecans (1/8 cup, roasted and chopped)

Chicken (1/8 cup, cooked and pulled)

**Directions:**

Heat 1 cup oil in a saucepan. While the oil is heating, whisk the eggs with soy sauce, and chicken. Your eggs should be filled with air bubbles. Once the oil is hot, pour the egg mix in the center of oil. Cook for 30 seconds or until bubbly and puffy. Flip the omelet and cook for 30 seconds more. Once the egg is golden brown remove from the oil and place onto a plate lined with paper towels. Top with arugula, chopped peppers, and chopped pecans. Serve and enjoy.

**Nutritional Information per Serving:**

Calories: 357.2; Total Fat: 3.4 g; Carbs: 42.7 g; Protein: 41.8 g;

# Day 3 – Lunch: Creamy Cauliflower Soup

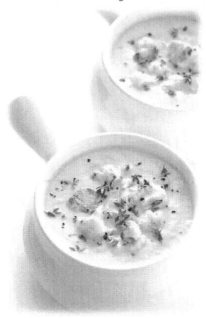

*Serves: 6*

**Time: 30 minutes**

**Ingredients:**

14oz. cauliflower heat, cut into florets

5oz. watercress

7oz. spinach, thawed

cups chicken stock

¼ cup ghee

Salt and pepper – 1 tsp. each to taste

1 onion, chopped

2 garlic cloves, crushed

## Directions:

Grease Dutch oven with ghee, place over medium-high heat and add onion and garlic. Cook until browned and stir cauliflower florets. Cook for 5 minutes. Add spinach and water cress and cook for 2 minutes or until just wilted, pour in vegetable stock and bring to boil.

Cook until cauliflower is crisp-tender and stir in the coconut milk. Season with salt and pepper and remove from the heat. Allow cooling and puree the soup in Vitamix until creamy. Strain and serve immediately.

## Nutritional Information per Serving:

Calories: 105; Total Fat: 8 g; Carbs: 6 g; Protein: 4 g;

# Day 3 – Dinner: Brown Stewed Pork

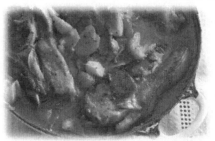

*Serves: 3-4*

**Time: 1 hour**

**Ingredients**

Thyme (1 sprig)

Bay Leaf (1 dry)

Cloves (2, whole)

Kitchen twine

Pork (2lbs, trimmed)

Sea salt and pepper (1 tsp each)

Vegetable oil (1/2 Cup)

Onion (1, small, diced)

Carrot (1, small, diced)

Celery (1 stalk, diced)

Tomato Paste (1 Tbsp.)

White Wine (1 Cup, dry)

Pork Stock (3 Cups)

Parsley (3 Tbsp., chopped)

## Directions

Create a bouquet garni by tying your cheesecloth with the thyme, rosemary, cloves, and bay leaf cloves inside then secure it with a piece of twine. Use a piece of paper towel to remove the excess moisture from the pork pieces in a patting motion. Season with salt and pepper. Heat the oil in your Dutch oven pot until it begins to smoke. Set your pork to brown on all sides. Remove the pork pieces from the heat and set aside. In the pot, you took the pork from, pour in the carrots, onion, and celery then add salt to season. Sauté for about 8 minutes or until completely soft. Mix in the tomato paste to the carrot mixture in the pot and add browned pork. Pour in the white wine and allow it to cook until the liquid is reduced by half.

Pour in the 2 cups of the stock along with the bouquet garni and allow boiling. Cover the pot, set the heat to low and simmer until the meat is literally falling off the bone when lifted. Ensure that the liquid is about ¾ way up the pork by checking on it in 15-minute intervals. When the meat has cooked remove the pork from the pot and plate in preparation to serve. Remove and discard the kitchen twine and the bouquet garni. Use the juices from the pot to pour over the pork pieces. Serve and Enjoy!

## Nutritional Information per Serving:

Calories: 120; Total Fat: 6.81 g; Carbs: 0 g; Protein: 13.62 g;

# Day 4 – Breakfast: Leek & Mushroom Frittata

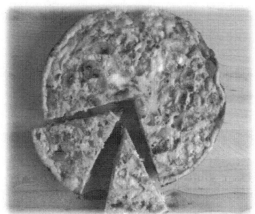

**Servings: 4 ½**

**Time: 30 minutes**

**Ingredients**

Mushroom (4 cups, shitake, sautéed until softened)

Eggs (6, large)

Garlic (1 clove, chopped fine)

Fontina Cheese (1/4 cup, grated)

Thyme (1 tbsp., chopped)

Skim Milk (1 cup, evaporated)

Leek (1, finely diced, sautéed until softened)

Olive oil (1 tsp)

Salt (1/4 tsp.)

Pepper (1/4 tsp.)

Cooking spray (enough to coat pan)

## Directions

Preheat oven to 375°F. In a medium bowl combine your mushrooms and leeks with half of your salt and pepper and olive oil. Spray a pie dish (9 inches) and spoon in your mushroom and leeks spreading to cover the entire bottom of the pie dish. In a bowl mix eggs, garlic, thyme, milk, pepper, and salt then pour mixture on top the mushrooms and leeks in your pie dish. Top evenly with fontina cheese. Allow to bake until puffy and golden in color (about 30 minutes). Allow to cool slightly, serve and enjoy.

## Nutritional Information per Serving:

Calories: 300; Total Fat: 21 g; Carbs: 9 g; Protein: 18 g;

# Day 4 – Lunch: Rustic Ragu with Pork

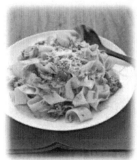

*Serves: 3-4*

**Time: 2 hour**

**Ingredients**

Pork (4 lbs.)

Salt

Pepper

Olive Oil (2 Tbsp.)

Onions (2, large, finely minced)

Tomato Paste (1/4 Cup)

Garlic (4 Cloves, minced)

Lemon Water (1 Cup, Dry)

Plum Tomatoes, (2 (796ml) Cans, Italian, crushed)

Star Anise Pods (two)

Bay Leaf (one)

Cooked Polenta

Parmesan Cheese (Shredded)

## Directions

Trim and discard the excess fat from the top of the roast. Remove the excess liquid from it by patting it dry then proceed to season it with salt and pepper. On medium setting heat the oil in a large Dutch oven. Now, for 3 to 4 minutes per side char the pork, or char it until browned on every side, before transferring it off to a platter.

Set your oven to preheat at 250F and as it does, add your seasoning of onions and tomato paste, occasionally stirring for 10 minutes or until the onion gets very soft. After this, garlic can be added while continuing to cooking for a minute or two. Add lemon water while stirring and watching for and putting back in any browned bits that are left in the pan. Immediately after, add the crushed tomatoes and tomato juice. Now, put back the roast into the pot and bring the mixture to a boil now by setting the heat to high.

The bay leaf and star anise should be wrapped in a cheesecloth pouch, dipped into the sauce and the pot covered. Move the pot now to your preheated oven for cooking for 3 hours. By this time your meat should be tender, falling away from its bone, at which time you may discard the bay leaf and star anise. Serve and enjoy.

## Nutritional Information per Serving:

Calories: 310; Total Fat: 5 g; Carbs: 57 g; Protein: 7 g;

# Day 4 – Dinner: Root Beer Ribs

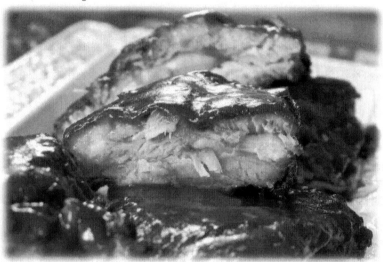

*Serves: 3 – 4*

**Time: 2 ½ hr.**

**Ingredients:**

Pork spare ribs (2 lbs.)

For the rub: Salt (1 tsp) Pepper (1 tsp) Spicy Hungarian paprika (1 tsp)

For the braise:
Large red onion, minced (1)
Section ginger, peeled, minced (1")
Cumin, crushed (1 tsp)

Spicy Hungarian paprika (1/4 tsp)
Bay leaves (3)
Cinnamon (1/4 tsp)
Root beer (1 bottle, 12 ounces)
Beef or chicken broth (1 cup)
Rosemary (2 sprigs)
Thyme (3 sprigs)

## Directions:

Set your oven to preheat to 275F. As well your large Dutch oven should be heated over a high fire. Your rib back should be rubbed in with salt, pepper, and your spicy paprika mix. Sear the ribs all over using a cooking tong until it gets to a good golden brown. Now remove your ribs to a plate. Your Dutch oven should be cleared of all the oil now but leave behind 2 tablespoons where onion should be added to medium-high heat until soft and the edges become brown. Return your ribs to the pot, including with it all the braise ingredients and boil the entire mixture. For a little while, cover before placing in the oven.

While in the oven and turning the ribs halfway through, braise for about 2 1/2 – 3 hours before removing from the oven. A large skillet should be placed on low heat for which you will now place your ribs. For the Dutch oven place your burner on high heat and remove the bay leaves. Boil the sauce down in here for approximately 20 minutes until you get to the desired thickness. Glaze your ribs with a bit of the sauce while stirring it.

You may finally slice your ribs nicely and smother it with sauce. Serve and enjoy over polenta, rice, or potatoes.

## Nutritional Information per Serving:

Calories: 490; Total Fat: 21 g; Carbs: 61 g; Protein: 12 g;

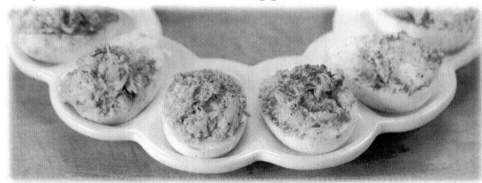

*Serves: 12*

**Time: 15 minutes**

**Ingredients**

Eggs (24, large, hard-boiled, peeled and halved)

Crab (12 oz., fresh, small diced)

Mayonnaise (1/3 cup)

Sour Cream (1/3 cup)

Lemon Juice (2 tsp.)

Tabasco Sauce (1 ½ tsp.)

Garlic Powder (1/2 tsp.)

Parsley (1 ½ tbsp., chopped)

Tarragon (1 ½ tbsp., fresh, chopped)

Tarragon (24 sprigs)

Salt & Pepper (2 tsp. ea.)

Paprika (2 tsp.)

## Directions

Scoop out the yolk of the eggs into a medium bowl and mix well with all the ingredients except for your egg whites and paprika. Add one tablespoon of your yolk mixture into each egg white half and sprinkle with paprika. Serve immediately or refrigerate until you are ready to serve.

## Nutritional Information per Serving:

Calories: 64; Total Fat: 4 g; Carbs: 1 g; Protein: 5 g;

# Day 5 – Lunch: Coconut Mushroom Soup

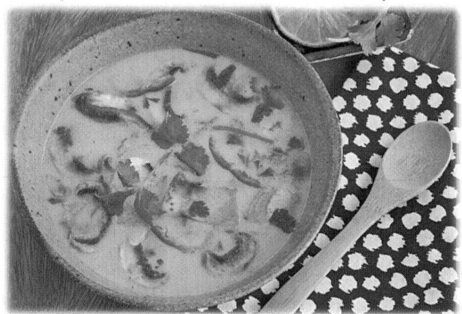

*Serves: 3*

**Time: 25 minutes**

**Ingredients**

1 cup mushrooms, sliced

1 cup coconut milk

1 onion, sliced

1 cup chicken broth

4-5 garlic cloves, minced

½ teaspoon black pepper

¼ teaspoon salt

1 tablespoon oil

## Directions

Heat oil in a saucepan, add onion and garlic cloves, cook for 1 minute. Add all mushroom and fry for 5 minutes. Add chicken broth, coconut milk, salt, pepper and mix well. Leave to cook on low heat for 15 minutes. Transfer to serving bowls. Serve and enjoy.

## Nutritional Information per Serving:

Calories: 180; Total Fat: 2 g; Carbs: 7 g; Protein: 3 g;

# Day 5 – Dinner: Beef Stew

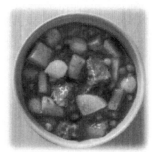

*Serves: 3-4*

**Time: 2 hours**

**Ingredients:**

Onion (1, small, diced)

Carrot (1, small, diced)

Celery (1 stalk, diced)

Thyme (1 sprig)

Bay Leaf (1 dry)

Cloves (2, whole)

Beef Stock (3 Cups)

Stew Beef (2lbs, trimmed, diced)

Sea salt and pepper (1 tsp each)

Vegetable oil (1/2 Cup)

Tomato Paste (1 Tbsp.)

White Wine (1 Cup, dry)

Parsley (3 Tbsp., chopped)

Lemon Zest (1 Tbsp.)

## Directions:

Create a bouquet garni by tying your cheesecloth with the thyme, rosemary, cloves, and bay leaf cloves inside then secure it with a piece of twine. Use a piece of paper towel to remove the excess moisture from the beef pieces in a patting motion. Season with salt and pepper. Heat the oil in your Dutch oven pot until it begins to smoke. Place the beef to brown on all sides. Remove the beef from the heat and set aside.

In the pot, you took the beef pieces from, pour in the carrots, onion, and celery then add salt to season. Sauté for about 8 minutes or until completely soft. Mix in the tomato paste to the carrot mixture in the pot and add browned beef. Pour in the white wine and allow it to cook until the liquid is reduced by half. Pour in the 2 cups of the beef stock along with the bouquet garni and allow boiling. Cover the pot, set the heat to low and simmer until the meat is literally falling off the bone when lifted. Ensure that the liquid is about ¾ way up the shank by checking on it in 15-minute intervals. When the meat has cooked remove the beef from the pot and plate in preparation to serve. Remove and discard the kitchen twine and the bouquet garni. Use the juices from the pot to pour over the beef pieces. Serve and Enjoy!

## Nutritional Information per Serving:

Calories: 209; Total Fat: 5.9 g; Carbs: 21.77 g; Protein: 16.98 g;

# Day 6 – Breakfast: Scrambled Eggs with Smoked Salmon

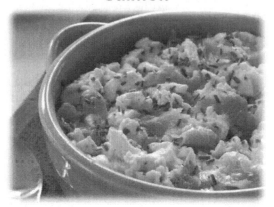

*Serving: 1*

**Time: 6 minutes**

**Ingredients:**

Eggs (2)

Smoked Salmon (1/8 cup, finely diced)

Heavy cream (1 tsp)

Butter (1 tsp)

Salt and pepper (1 tsp, or to taste)

Water (1 tsp)

**Directions:**

In a small bowl add the eggs, water, and heavy cream then mix around using a fork. Over low heat melt the butter in a skillet. Pour the egg mixture into the skillet. Stir constantly. About a minute in add in your salmon and continue to stir once the egg is set and still moist. Add the salt and pepper while it is on the plate.

**Nutritional Information per Serving:**

Calories: 200; Total Fat: 13.3 g; Carbs: 2.3 g; Protein: 16.7 g;

# Day 6 – Lunch: Chicken Curry Stew

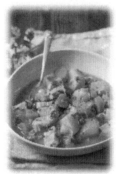

*Serves: 4*

**Time: 4 hours 15 minutes**

**Ingredients:**

5 chicken tights

5 chicken drumsticks

1 tablespoon Worcestershire sauce

14oz. can coconut milk

½ cup chicken stock

2 tablespoons fish sauce

2 tablespoons brown sugar

4 tablespoons red curry paste

1 tablespoon lemon juice

2 limes, juiced and zested

1 tablespoon olive oil

½ teaspoon Salt

¼ teaspoon Pepper

## Directions:

Turn on the slow cooker. Heat the oil in a skillet over medium-high heat. Season the chicken and cook in the oil until browned on all sides. Remove and place in heated slow cooker. Cook the curry paste in the same skillet for 1-2 minutes or until fragrant.

Add the Worcestershire sauce, brown sugar, and lemon juice. Cook until the sugar is melted. Pour in the stock, coconut milk, fish sauce, lime juice, and zest. Give it all a good stir and pour into the slow cooker. Cover and cook on high for 4 hours (or on low for 8 hours). Serve

## Nutritional Information per Serving:

Calories: 387; Total Fat: 16.2 g; Carbs: 26.3 g; Protein: 35.3 g;

# Day 6 – Dinner: Vegetarian Curry

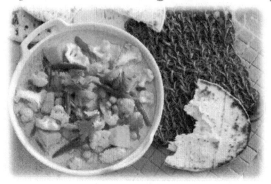

*Serves: 4*

**Time: 40 hours 35 minutes**

**Ingredients:**

16oz. extra firm tofu drained and cut into cubes

1 eggplant, chopped

14oz. can coconut milk

1 tablespoon palm sugar

¼ cup Thai green paste

1 ½ cups sliced bell pepper

1 onion, sliced

½ teaspoon turmeric

2 cup broccoli flowers

¾ cup peas

1 tablespoon minced ginger

1 cup vegetable broth

 Salt, to taste

## Directions:

In a Dutch oven, combine the milk, curry paste, sugar, turmeric and vegetable broth. Season with salt to taste. Add the onion, bell pepper, and eggplant. Cook on high for 3-4 hours. Meanwhile, heat some oil in a skillet over medium-high heat. Add the tofu and cook until golden on all sides. Place aside. During the last 30 minutes, add the tofu and broccoli. Allow the curry to cook for the remaining 30 minutes and serve after.

## Nutritional Information per Serving:

Calories: 307; Total Fat: 19.9 g; Carbs: 19.1 g; Protein: 11.1 g;

# Day 7 – Breakfast: Eggs, Ham & Pineapple Pizza

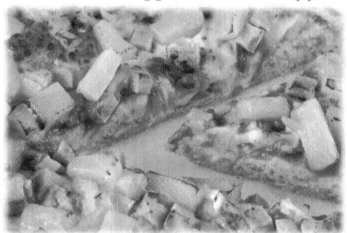

*Serves: 12*

**Time: 50 minutes**

**Ingredients:**

Ham (10 slices)

Pineapple (10 slices)

Eggs (12, beaten)

Salt and Pepper (1 tbs. or to taste)

Refrigerated crescent roll dough (2 packages)

Salsa (1/2 cup)

Cheddar cheese (2 cups, shredded)

**Directions:**

On medium heat cook, the ham in a skillet for five minutes on both sides or until it is browned evenly. Drain on a paper towel. Scrambled the egg for 5 minutes or till it is no longer wet. Season with the salt and pepper. Preheat the oven to 350 degrees F. Let the crescent roll fit the bottom of a 9x13 baking dish. Bake, the dough for 10 minutes or until it, is golden brown. Sprinkle the salsa all over the baked dough, top with the scrambled egg, then crumbled the ham on top, chop the pineapple slices and spread it everywhere then add the cheese. Bake for ten minutes or till the cheese has melted. Let it cool for ten minutes before cutting into it. Serve and enjoy.

**Nutritional Information per Serving:**

Calories: 204; Total Fat: 10.6 g; Carbs: 13.5 g; Protein: 13.6 g;

# Day 7 – Lunch: Brussel Sprouts & Bacon Egg Salad

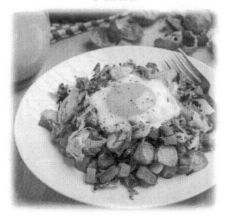

**Serves: 6**

**Time: 30m + chilling time**

**Ingredients:**

Brussel Sprouts (4 cups, roasted and shaved)

Hard-boiled eggs (4, peeled, and chopped finely)

Bacon (1/4 cup, baked and chopped)

Basil Mayo (¼ cup)

Celery (2 stalks, diced)

Red onion (4 G.O, chopped)

Sour cream (1/4 cup)

Apple Cider Vinegar (2 tablespoons)

White sugar (1 teaspoon)

Salt and black pepper (to taste)

## Directions:

Place all ingredients in a large bowl and mix until it is thoroughly combined. Chill for at least 1 hour before serving. Serve and enjoy.

## Nutritional Information per Serving:

Calories: 351.6; Total Fat: 22 g; Carbs: 23.8 g; Protein: 16 g;

# Day 7 – Dinner: Zoodles & Meatballs

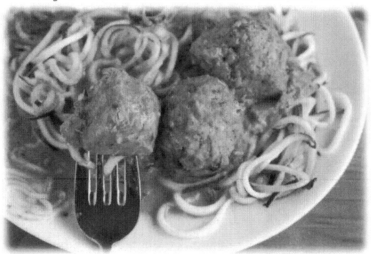

*Serves: 4*

Time: 45 minutes

**Ingredients**

2 oz. beef mince

2 large zucchinis

1 onion, chopped

1 teaspoon cayenne pepper

½ teaspoon chili powder

1 cup tomato sauce

2 tablespoons gram flour

2 tablespoons olive oil

½ teaspoon garlic paste

1 teaspoon cumin powder

1 teaspoon cinnamon powder

2-3 garlic cloves, minced

¼ teaspoon salt

2 tablespoons lemon juice

1 tablespoon butter

## Directions

Preheat oven to 355 degrees F and place parchment sheet on a baking tray. In a bowl combine beef mince, gram flour, salt, chili powder, cumin powder, cinnamon powder, garlic paste, and onion, mix. Make round balls and place in baking dish. Bake for 20-25 minutes. In a sauce pan add garlic cloves and sauté for 1 minute. Stir, in tomato sauce and season with cayenne pepper and some salt. Cook for 5-6 minutes.

Add baked meatballs and toss carefully to combine. Melt butter in a pan and sauté zucchini for 1-2 minutes and drizzle lemon juice on top. Transfer zoodles in serving dish and top with meatballs. Enjoy.

## Nutritional Information per Serving:

Calories: 325; Total Fat: 15 g; Carbs: 25 g; Protein: 25 g;

# Bonus Dessert: Sugar-free Melon & Berry Sorbet

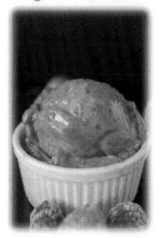

*Serves: 6*

**Time: 5 minutes**

**Ingredients:**

4 ½ cups ice cubes, crushed

½lb Melon, cubed

½ cup Mixed berries

1 tablespoon grated orange zest

2 tablespoons honey

**Directions:**

Place all ingredients in a blender. Blend the ingredients for 30 seconds. Serve immediately.

**Nutritional Information per Serving:**

Calories: 97.5; Total Fat: 0.7 g; Carbs: 24.2 g; Protein: 1 g;

# Bonus Dessert: Sugar-free Blackberry Cheesecake

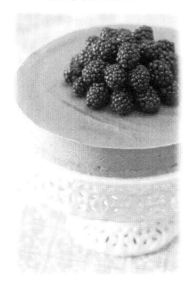

*Serves: 4*

**Time: 30 minutes**

**Ingredients**

1 cup blackberry puree

1 teaspoon vanilla extract

3 cups cream cheese

½ cup whipped cream

1 cup blackberries

2 tablespoons butter, melted

3 egg whites

1/2 cup condense milk

2 packages of graham crackers, crumbled

## Directions

Preheat oven to 350 degrees. Beat egg whites until fluffy. In separate bowl beat cream cheese until fuzzy. Now add in it whipped cream, whipped egg whites, blackberry puree, butter, condensed milk, vanilla and folded it. Spread crumbled crackers into greased round baking pan and press well. Pour cheese mixture and set it with a spatula evenly.

Bake for 25-30 minutes. When the cake is made, place it in the freezer for 20 minutes. Top with blackberries and serve.

## Nutritional Information per Serving:

Calories: 334; Total Fat: 32 g; Carbs: 5 g; Protein: 9 g;

# Conclusion

Congratulations on making it all the way to the end! This shows that you are serious about taking the next step of your intermittent fasting journey! I will end by reminding you of the last tip we covered to stay on track, and that's to remember to maintain realistic goals.

As much as we would like to believe that you will be the next great miracle of intermittent fasting, it is better to keep your expectations as realistic as possible. Sure, intermittent fasting, if done correctly, has the potential to assist you in your weight loss journey, increase your body's sensitivity to insulin, and regulate the rate in which your body secretes growth hormones, which are all wonderful benefits. However, it is important that you also keep in mind that intermittent fasting is just one aspect of the many things you will need to adjust in your life to achieve success in your body's overall health. You will also need to adjust your overall level of activity, amount of sleep, stress levels and it will take time.

Once again, I want to thank you for allowing me to guide you along this journey and wish you all the success possible on your intermittent fasting journey. Don't forget to leave me a positive review if you like what you read. Until next time, happy fasting!

Dear Reader,
Thank you for buying and reading my book!
If you like it, please, leave a review. It is important for me and
my future books.
Just scan this qr code and you can leave a review

Or just type this link –

**https://www.amazon.com/review/create-review?ie=UTF8&asin=B079MH7WSP#**

**Thank you!**
**I really appreciate it!**

Made in the USA
San Bernardino, CA
16 March 2018